BEGINNER GUIDE TO WATER AEROBICS FOR FITNESS

Master Aquatic Exercises, Aqua Workouts, And Pool Fitness Techniques For Weight Loss, Cardiovascular Health, And Muscle Toning

MALCOLM KASHTON

All rights reserved. Except for brief quotations included in critical reviews and certain other noncommercial uses allowed by copyright law, no part of this book may be reproduced, distributed, or transmitted in any form or by any means, electronic or mechanical, including photocopying, recording, or by any information storage and retrieval system, without the author's prior written permission.

Despite their best efforts, the author and publisher disclaim all liability for any mistakes or omissions in the information included in this book, as well as for any damages that may arise from using it.

DISCLAIMER

This book contains information that is solely meant to be used for educational and informative reasons. This includes training regimens, game strategy, and fitness recommendations. Despite having taken every precaution to guarantee the correctness and completeness of the material provided, the author disclaims all express and implied warranties and representations regarding the content's suitability, timeliness, reliability, or accuracy for any purpose.

This book's content is not meant to be a replacement for expert medical advice, diagnosis, or care. When in doubt about a medical problem, never hesitate to consult your doctor or another trained healthcare professional. Never ignore medical advice from professionals or put off getting it because of something you've read in this book.

The material provided here and how you utilize it are not the responsibility of the author or publisher. You bear full responsibility for any reliance you make on the information contained in this book. The publisher and author disclaim all liability for any loss or damage resulting from using this book, including but not limited to indirect or consequential loss or damage, or any loss or damage from losing data or profits.

All references in this book to particular goods, services, or organizations are made for informative purposes only and do not imply endorsement or recommendation on the part of the publisher or author.

You acknowledge that there is no responsibility for any harm or injury that may arise from utilizing the material in this book, and that you will hold the author and publisher harmless by reading and using it. You alone are in charge of your own health and wellbeing, so you should apply any advice or suggestions from this book with caution and good judgment.

Table Of Contents

ABOUT THE BOOK

"Water Aerobics for Fitness" is an invaluable reference that completely investigates the world of water aerobics, presenting a wealth of information and practical insights for anyone wishing to better their fitness levels through aquatic exercises. The book opens with a perceptive introduction that highlights the value of water aerobics and gives readers a sense of the author's experience. The objective of the book is clearly described, highlighting its role in creating comprehensive well-being.

The book digs into the essential components of water aerobics, revealing its definition, historical evolution, and the compelling reasons behind choosing it as a workout regimen. The book walk readers through the steps of getting started, making sure they are safe, choosing the best pool, and comprehending the necessary equipment for a good practice of water aerobics.

Basic skills are clarified, creating a solid basis for readers to embark on their fitness adventure in the water.

As the book develops, it covers a varied range of themes, including warm-up exercises, aerobic workouts, strength training, flexibility, and balance routines adapted for the aquatic environment. A wide range of readers can find the book inclusive and accessible because special consideration is given to accommodating varied demographics, including the elderly, expectant mothers, and people with impairments.

The advanced techniques chapter introduces readers to high-intensity interval training (HIIT) and advanced water aerobics maneuvers, empowering them to upgrade their workout routines. The book also incorporates dietary advice and stresses the significance of staying hydrated when engaging in aquatic activity. This extensive book is interwoven with ideas for recovery and cooling down, addressing frequent problems, and mixing water aerobics with other fitness routines.

 The essential elements of developing a sustainable routine are covered, and readers are urged to make long-term plans, establish reasonable objectives, and maintain motivation throughout their fitness journey. "Water Aerobics for Fitness" is a comprehensive resource that encourages people to embrace water aerobics as a fun and transformative way to reach and maintain optimal health and fitness in addition to providing education.

CHAPTER ONE

OVERVIEW OF WATER AEROBICS FOR FITNESS

WHAT WATER AEROBICS OFFERS

A well-liked and successful form of exercise that combines cardiovascular fitness with the special qualities of water is called water aerobics. This water exercise has a plethora of benefits, making it an intriguing option for anyone seeking a low-impact yct tough workout.

One of the key advantages of water aerobics is its ability to deliver a full-body workout while minimizing stress on the joints and muscles.

For people with arthritis, joint discomfort, or other mobility problems, water is a great option because of its buoyancy, which lessens the strain on weight-bearing joints.

KNOWING WATER AEROBICS

Recognizing how water resistance enhances the training experience is essential to understanding the notion of water aerobics. Resistance rises as people travel through the water, requiring more work and energy than in conventional land-based exercises. This increased resistance helps to increase general endurance and stamina in addition to strengthening muscles. Both novices and seasoned exercise enthusiasts can benefit from water aerobics because it can be tailored to accommodate different fitness levels.

CONCEPT AND DEFINITION

The incorporation of aerobic workouts in a water environment is what defines water aerobics. Participants engage in rhythmic motions and exercises intended to increase heart rate and improve cardiovascular fitness, usually in a shallow pool. To target different muscle groups, water aerobics sessions frequently incorporate a variety of exercises such as arm movements, jumping jacks, running, and water walking. Apart from its cardiovascular advantages, water aerobics integrates resistance training components that enhance strength and flexibility.

WATER AEROBICS' PAST

Examining the past of water aerobics shows how the fitness phenomena have developed throughout time. Water aerobics, which started in the late 20th century, became well-liked as a fun and safe substitute for conventional land-based aerobics. Because of its gentleness, it was first mostly utilized as a rehabilitation aid for people healing from injuries. Water aerobics became a part of popular exercise regimens over time due to its favorable effects and wide spectrum of participants. It is now a standard feature in a lot of fitness centers and public swimming pools worldwide.

WHY GO FOR WATER AEROBICS AS A FITNESS OPTION?

The decision to choose water aerobics for fitness is based on its many benefits. Water aerobics is suitable for people of all ages and fitness levels due to its low-impact nature. It offers a secure and practical means of maintaining an active lifestyle, making it especially appealing to those suffering from osteoporosis, arthritis, or recuperating from injuries. Water's buoyancy further lowers the chance of damage while yet providing a strenuous workout that hits several muscle groups at once. The social component of water aerobics sessions adds to their allure by encouraging a sense of camaraderie and solidarity among participants. Whether you're looking for a fun and social workout, toning your muscles, or better cardiovascular health, selecting water aerobics as your fitness option promotes a comprehensive approach to physical well-being.

CHAPTER TWO

BEGINNING

SAFETY MEASURES

As with any aquatic activity, water aerobics is an activity in which safety must always come first. To ensure that participants are safe, it is important to follow some safety measures before beginning a water aerobics exercise. First and foremost, before participating in water aerobics, people with pre-existing medical concerns should speak with their healthcare practitioners to make sure the activity is appropriate for them. A qualified teacher must also be present during all sessions to mentor participants and offer support when required.

Moreover, adequate hydration is essential for water aerobics since the buoyancy of the water might mask the feeling of perspiration. It is important to remind participants to stay hydrated by drinking water regularly. It's also essential to have enough warm-up and cool-down times to avoid injuries and improve flexibility. To prevent collisions, participants should be encouraged to pay attention to their surroundings, particularly in crowded pool areas. Enough signage that displays the rules, emergency exits, and the depth of the pool is necessary to guarantee that everyone is aware of the safety procedures.

SELECTING THE APPROPRIATE POOL

Choosing the right pool is essential to having a good water aerobics experience. The success of the workout can be greatly impacted by selecting the correct pool because they are available in a variety of sizes, depths, and temperatures. Water aerobics works best in a pool that is 3 to 5 feet deep because it strikes a balance between buoyancy and resistance. Participants should be able to comfortably swim in water that is typically between 82 and 88 degrees Fahrenheit.

Apart from the physical characteristics of the pool, the facility's upkeep and cleanliness are also quite important. In addition to guaranteeing a clean atmosphere, a well-kept pool lowers the chance of trips and falls. When choosing a pool for water aerobics sessions, accessible restrooms and changing areas are also crucial considerations.

EQUIPMENT NEEDED

Although the resistance offered by the water is the main source of difficulty in water aerobics, adding the appropriate equipment can improve the workout's efficiency. Swim noodles, buoyancy belts, and water dumbbells are examples of basic equipment. While flotation belts provide buoyancy, enabling participants to concentrate on particular exercises without worrying about sinking, water dumbbells add resistance to movements, aiding in the strengthening and toning of muscles. Swim noodles are useful for a variety of activities that improve stability and balance.

For the comfort and safety of participants, appropriate swimwear is also needed, including swim caps and goggles. The footwear that is worn is equally important; water shoes protect participants' feet and offer traction on pool surfaces. Setting up the equipment for water aerobics classes should take practical considerations such as having enough room for personal items and a sound system for music if desired.

FUNDAMENTAL WATER AEROBICS METHODS

A range of exercises aimed at increasing strength, flexibility, and cardiovascular fitness are included in water aerobics techniques. To gradually increase heart rate, warm-up exercises usually entail marching or running in place. Cardiovascular workouts that increase stamina and burn calories include jumping jacks, jogging, and water walking.

In water aerobics, resistance training entails working against muscle groups with the water. Exercises like leg lifts, torso twists, and water dumbbell curls can help achieve this.

Range-of-motion exercises also aid in improving flexibility; for example, arm circles and leg swings encourage joint mobility.

Exercises for cooling down are crucial for reducing heart rate gradually and avoiding muscle discomfort. Flexibility may be increased and muscles can be relaxed with simple stretches like sitting leg stretches and toe touches. To get the most out of water aerobics, participants should be urged to concentrate on regulated movements, appropriate breathing, and keeping good posturc throughout the exercise.

CHAPTER THREE

EXERCISES FOR THE HEART

SWIMMING JOGGING

Cardiovascular workouts comprise a wide variety of activities intended to improve endurance, heart health, and general fitness. Aqua jogging is one of the most popular and least impactful of these. By simulating running in the water, aqua jogging provides resistance that works for different muscle groups.

This buoyant workout is good for people who have joint problems or are recovering from accidents since it lessens the strain on joints.

SWIMMING IN THE WATER

Another effective cardiovascular exercise that may be done in an aquatic setting is water walking. Due to its buoyancy, swimming is a moderate and accessible activity that can be done by people of varying fitness levels. People can tone their muscles, improve their balance, and increase their cardiovascular endurance by walking against the resistance of the water. Those looking for a low-impact substitute for conventional land-based activities will find that walking on the water is very advantageous.

FLOWING WATER

Adding water running to your training regimen adds a dynamic and difficult exercise. Running in a pool increases cardiovascular exertion and promotes muscle engagement and calorie burning due to the increased resistance of the water.

Running in the water is a great way to add some variety to your cardiovascular training regimen, and it also helps people become more stable and strong in their core as they move through the water.

AEROBICS IN WATER EXERCISES

A thorough and entertaining approach to developing cardiovascular fitness while utilizing the advantages of water resistance is through water aerobics programs. These workouts usually consist of a sequence of cardiovascular exercises done in an aquatic setting, like jumping jacks, leg lifts, and arm movements.

A full-body workout that targets various muscle groups and improves cardiovascular health is what water aerobics offers.

Because of the buoyancy of the water, athletes must use their muscles more efficiently, adding a difficulty element.

There are a variety of cardiovascular exercise alternatives available with aqua jogging, water walking, water running, and water aerobics exercises. Because the water environment offers a special combination of buoyancy and resistance, people with different physical conditions and fitness levels can perform these exercises. These water-based exercises improve cardiovascular health and make working out more enjoyable when incorporated into a fitness program.

CHAPTER FOUR
WARM-UP ACTIVITIES

THE VALUE OF WARM-UP

Any fitness regimen needs to include warm-up activities since they act as a prelude that progressively raises heart rate, improves blood flow to the muscles, and loosens up joints. The benefits of warm-up exercises include lowering the risk of injury and enhancing performance by preparing the body for more demanding physical activity. Following a suitable warm-up regimen improves balance and coordination by activating the neuromuscular system and mentally preparing people for the physical exertion that lies ahead.

STRETCHING DYNAMICALLY IN WATER

A novel and useful method for preheating the body before participating in physical activity is dynamic stretching in the water. Water's buoyancy lessens the force on joints, making this a low impact but incredibly effective technique. Dynamic stretching includes smooth, deliberate motions that extend the range of motion of the muscles and joints. Stretching dynamically in the water adds resistance to the movements, making it a gentle but efficient technique to improve blood circulation and flexibility. As it reduces joint tension while maintaining joint mobility, this is especially advantageous for people with joint problems or those recovering from injuries.

EXERCISES FOR JOINT MOBILITY

Warm-up programs must include joint mobility exercises, which are designed to improve the range of motion in different joints throughout the body. These workouts focus on targeted joints such as the knees, ankles, shoulders, and hips through controlled movements. Exercises that increase joint lubrication, enhance synovial fluid circulation, and lessen stiffness are the goals of joint mobility. They also support appropriate movement patterns by improving kinesthetic awareness and proprioception.

For both athletes and fitness enthusiasts, including joint mobility exercises in a warm-up regimen, is crucial since it can improve overall functional capacity and lower the risk of problems associated with limited joint mobility.

Warm-up activities are crucial because they lay the groundwork for safe and productive physical activity. A novel and gentle method of warming up is dynamic stretching in water, which is especially helpful for people with joint issues. Conversely, joint mobility exercises aim to increase a particular joint's range of motion, increase general flexibility, and lower the risk of injury. Including these ideas in a thorough warm-up regimen can make a big difference in a person's general health and fitness.

CHAPTER FIVE

STRENGTH TRAINING IN THE WATER

ADVANTAGES OF RESISTANCE TO WATER

Building and sustaining muscle strength can be accomplished in a novel and efficient way with strength training in the water. There are several advantages to using water resistance training in strength training, including both therapeutic and physical benefits. One of the main advantages is the water's continuous resistance, which gives muscles something tough to work against. This resistance promotes healthy muscle development and lowers the chance of injury since it is more uniformly distributed over the whole range of motion.

Moreover, water resistance is easy on the joints, which makes it a great choice for people who have joint problems or are healing from accidents. Water's buoyancy lessens the force applied to the joints, reducing strain on the knees, hips, and other sensitive parts. This opens up the possibility of aquatic strength training to a wider group of people, including those suffering from musculoskeletal disorders like arthritis.

The natural cooling effect that water resistance offers while exercising is one of its main benefits. Water helps the body release heat, reducing overheating and enabling longer, more intense activities. In hotter climates or for people who have trouble staying warm during conventional land-based strength training, this can be especially helpful.

SIMPLE STRENGTH TRAINING

Simple strength training in the water can work a variety of muscle groups, providing a whole-body workout. Engaging in lower body exercises such as water walking or jogging can improve cardiovascular fitness and leg strength. When done in the water, leg lifts and kicks strengthen the core muscles, which enhances balance and stability.

The arms, shoulders, and chest can all be efficiently strengthened with arm workouts like resistance paddling or underwater push-ups.

Moreover, flexibility and range of motion can benefit from water-based strength training. In every workout, the resistance of the water promotes joint flexibility and decreases stiffness by encouraging a full range of motion. This can be especially helpful for people who want to increase their general level of mobility and stop their joints from degrading with age.

INCLUDING RESISTANCE INSTRUMENTS

Using resistance equipment to augment water-based strength training can give the exercise a new level of complexity. The resistance can be increased using water dumbbells or resistance bands, giving the muscles an even greater strain. Exercises like triceps extensions, lateral raises, and bicep curls can be performed more creatively with these instruments, increasing the workout's overall efficacy.

The workout is kept interesting and entertaining by the resistance tools, which also add variety to the regimen.

Strength training in the water has several advantages, from improved flexibility and cardiovascular fitness to stronger muscles and better joint protection. When modified for the aquatic environment, basic strength exercises offer a comprehensive workout that targets many muscle groups. Water-based strength training becomes much more effective when resistance tools are included, which makes it a flexible and affordable choice for people of all fitness levels. The water offers a dynamic environment for reaching and maintaining optimal physical health, whether you're looking for low-impact training or a demanding strength-building regimen.

CHAPTER SIX
ADAPTABILITY AND EQUILIBRIUM
IN THE WATER, STRETCHING

Balance and flexibility are essential for overall physical health since they greatly increase mobility and lower the chance of injury. To solve these difficulties, several creative ways have been developed; one noteworthy one is stretching in water. Using the buoyancy and resistance of water, this aquatic stretching technique creates a special environment for increasing flexibility. Water immersion is a great alternative for people who have limited movement or are recovering from injuries since it reduces the strain on joints and muscles.

Stretching in the water is a dynamic and rehabilitative experience since the water's resistance tests your muscles at every point of motion. Because of the inherent buoyancy of water, longer stretches can be performed without putting too much pressure on the body due to the reduced gravitational pull. This sort of stretching is not only helpful for building flexibility but also serves as a low-impact workout, making it accessible to a wide range of folks, including the elderly and those with joint concerns.

YOGA IN THE POOL

Yoga in the pool is another new approach that blends the principles of conventional yoga with the benefits of water immersion. The buoyancy of the water gives an element of support to yoga positions, enabling practitioners to explore deeper stretches and poses with lower pressure on the joints. Poolside yoga programs generally feature a blend of classic yoga postures, breathing exercises, and meditation, improving both physical and emotional well-being.

BALANCE EXERCISES

Balance exercises have a critical role in strengthening stability and minimizing falls, especially as persons age or experience certain physical problems.

Traditional balance exercises can be enhanced and diversified when performed in water, giving an extra degree of challenge. The resistance of water forces the engagement of core muscles and requires enhanced coordination to maintain balance. Activities such as standing on one leg, leg swings, or even basic weight changes become more dynamic and difficult when completed in the aquatic environment.

Engaging in balance exercises in the water not only increases physical stability but also fosters increased proprioception—the body understands of its position in space. This heightened awareness correlates to greater overall balance, minimizing the likelihood of falls and injuries. Moreover, the supporting nature of water makes these exercises accessible to persons with varied levels of fitness, accommodating those who may find traditional balance exercises on land too demanding.

The concepts of stretching in water, yoga in the pool, and balance exercises are unique techniques to promote flexibility and balance. These aquatic sports harness the unique features of water, such as buoyancy and resistance, to create a supportive environment for persons of all ages and fitness levels. Incorporating these strategies into a regular training regimen not only contributes to increased physical health but also adds a refreshing and pleasurable dimension to the goal of flexibility and balance.

CHAPTER SEVEN
SPECIAL POPULATIONS
WATER AEROBICS FOR SENIORS

Water aerobics for seniors is a popular and efficient kind of exercise that offers several benefits for this unique demographic. Seniors often confront obstacles such as musculoskeletal pain, diminished flexibility, and balance issues. Water aerobics provides a low-impact setting, lowering stress on joints and making it a suitable workout alternative for older persons. The buoyancy of water helps sustain body weight, making activities easier and minimizing the danger of injury. Additionally, water resistance promotes muscle strength and cardiovascular fitness without putting excessive load on the body.

PRENATAL WATER WORKOUTS

Prenatal water workouts cater exclusively to pregnant individuals, acknowledging the unique requirements and concerns of new mothers. Engaging in water activities during pregnancy is a safe and pleasant method to keep active. The buoyancy of water lowers the impact on joints and the chance of falling, offering a soothing atmosphere for pregnant women. Prenatal water workouts focus on building strength, flexibility, and cardiovascular fitness while taking into consideration the changing body of the expectant woman. These workouts contribute to increased mood, reduced edema, and enhanced overall well-being during pregnancy.

ADAPTING EXERCISES FOR INDIVIDUALS WITH DISABILITIES

Adapting activities for individuals with disabilities is a crucial part of inclusive fitness training. It entails altering standard workouts to fit the unique demands of people with various disabilities. In the context of water-based activities, adjusting routines guarantees that those with impairments can enjoy the benefits of aquatic fitness.

This may include changing movements, providing additional assistance, or employing assistive technology to enhance participation. Adapted water workouts not only promote physical health but also contribute to social inclusion and enhanced mental well-being for those with disabilities, generating a sense of empowerment and community.

Water aerobics for the elderly, prenatal water workouts and adapted activities for those with impairments are all vital components of specialized fitness programs. These approaches prioritize the unique requirements and problems of these special populations, supporting total health and well-being. Whether it's giving a low-impact option for the elderly, a safe exercise alternative for pregnant women, or inclusive exercises for those with disabilities, these themes illustrate the necessity of personalizing fitness programs to accommodate varied needs and abilities.

CHAPTER EIGHT

ADVANCED METHODS

HIGH-INTENSITY INTERVAL TRAINING (HIIT)

High-Intensity Interval Training (HIIT) has garnered tremendous appeal in the arena of fitness for its efficiency in burning calories and boosting cardiovascular health. This advanced strategy involves alternating short bursts of intensive exercise with brief periods of rest or lower-intensity activity. The primary premise underlying HIIT is to force the body to perform at maximum capacity during high-intensity intervals, followed by a recovery phase that allows the heart rate to decrease somewhat before the next difficult session.

One of the key advantages of HIIT is its time efficiency, making it a popular choice for persons with busy schedules. Research indicates that HIIT can lead to considerable increases in aerobic and anaerobic fitness, as well as metabolic health. The intensive nature of the workout drives the body to burn calories not only during the exercise session but also in the post-exercise phase, known as the after burn effect or excess post-exercise oxygen consumption (EPOC).

However, it's vital to approach HIIT with caution, especially for novices or persons with certain health conditions. Proper warm-up and cool-down periods are crucial to prevent injuries, and participants should customize the intensity and duration of the intervals to their fitness levels. Consulting with a fitness professional or healthcare practitioner is essential before going on a HIIT program to ensure it corresponds with specific health objectives and conditions.

ADVANCED WATER AEROBICS MOVES

Water aerobics, traditionally considered a low-impact exercise, can be pushed to a more advanced level with the introduction of demanding movements. Advanced water aerobics techniques harness the resistance of the water to activate several muscle groups while reducing stress on the joints.

Such techniques include complicated leg lifts, scissor kicks, and dynamic arm movements that involve higher strength and coordination.

The buoyancy of water minimizes the impact on joints, making it a perfect environment for persons with arthritis or joint issues. Advanced water aerobics techniques may entail the use of specialized equipment such as water dumbbells, resistance gloves, or buoyancy belts to improve the workout. These gadgets provide resistance, requiring extra effort from the muscles to accomplish each movement.

The multidirectional resistance given by water necessitates a heightened awareness of balance and stability, contributing to better core strength. Additionally, the regular activation of muscles in water helps build cardiovascular endurance. Individuals searching for a demanding yet joint-friendly workout can benefit from including advanced water aerobics movements in their fitness routine.

CREATING CUSTOMIZED WORKOUTS

Customizing workouts is a fundamental aspect of achieving fitness goals that cater to individual needs, preferences, and capabilities. Advanced techniques in creating customized workouts involve a comprehensive understanding of factors such as fitness level, specific objectives, time constraints, and any existing health considerations. Tailoring a workout program ensures that it remains engaging, sustainable, and aligned with the individual's long-term fitness journey.

Advanced customization may involve periodization, a strategic approach that varies the intensity and volume of workouts over distinct periods to prevent plateaus and optimize performance. This could include alternating between strength-focused, hypertrophy-focused, and endurance-focused phases. Incorporating a variety of exercises that target different muscle groups and movement patterns helps achieve a well-rounded fitness routine.

CHAPTER NINE

CONSUMPTION AND DRINKING WATER

NUTRITION'S SIGNIFICANCE

Nutrition is essential for sustaining general health and well-being since it provides the building blocks for many body processes. Beyond just quelling hunger, nutrition is vital for giving our bodies the fuel they need and for supporting the growth, development, and healthy operation of our organs and systems. Every ingredient in a well-balanced diet—carbohydrates, proteins, fats, vitamins, and minerals—contributes to a different physiological process. For example, the main source of energy is carbohydrates, yet proteins are necessary for muscle growth and repair. Nutrient-dense fats are important for hormone production and cell structure, while vitamins and minerals help the immune system and maintain bone health, among other things.

Sufficient nutrition is especially important for athletes and anyone who exercises often. Athletes frequently need more energy, and depending on the kind, intensity, and length of their workouts, they may require different amounts of nutrients. In addition to improving performance, a healthy diet speeds up healing and lowers the chance of injury. Maintaining stamina, endurance, and mental clarity during physical activities depends on consuming the proper ratio of macronutrients to micronutrients.

HYDRATION TECHNIQUES FOR SWIMMING EXERCISE

It's equally important to stay hydrated, especially when doing water exercises or any other kind of physical activity. Water is necessary for several body processes, such as digestion, nutrition transport, and temperature regulation. The body loses water through sweat when exercising, so it's critical to be well-hydrated to avoid dehydration, which can cause cramps, exhaustion, and decreased performance.

Because some exercises include submersion in water, such as swimming or aqua aerobics, maintaining proper hydration becomes more difficult. Although perspiration may not be as noticeable to others, people nonetheless lose fluids by breathing and, to some extent, through absorbing water.

Hydration tactics for activity in the water need to balance the amount of water consumed with the possibility of fluid loss. Hydration is crucial before, during, and following the activity. Prehydrating makes it more likely that the body will begin an exercise session sufficiently hydrated. Even if they do not feel as thirsty as they would during other types of activity, people should nevertheless drink water often when exercising in the water. A tailored strategy for maintaining proper hydration involves tracking each person's rate of perspiration and modifying fluid intake accordingly. Electrolyte balance is also important because it helps maintain appropriate muscle function and prevents cramping, which is especially important for prolonged aquatic sports.

Anyone looking to maintain a healthy and active lifestyle must recognize the significance of diet and water. While adequate hydration is vital for maintaining energy levels and preventing dehydration during physical activity, including water exercise, sufficient nutrition supplies the building blocks for optimal biological function. Through conscientious dietary decisions and the application of efficient hydration techniques, people can improve their general health and performance in a range of physical activities.

CHAPTER TEN

RECOVERY AND COOLING DOWN

COOLING DOWN EXERCISES

Cooling down exercises are a crucial component of any workout routine, serving as a gradual transition from intense physical activity to a state of rest. These exercises typically involve low-intensity movements and stretches that help bring the heart rate back to its pre-exercise state.

Engaging in cooling-down exercises is essential for preventing muscle soreness and stiffness, as it allows the body to gradually return to its baseline state, reducing the risk of injury. These exercises may include gentle jogging, walking, or specific stretches targeting major muscle groups. Incorporating cooling-down exercises into a fitness regimen contributes to overall flexibility and joint mobility, fostering long-term physical well-bcing.

IMPORTANCE OF POST-WORKOUT RECOVERY

Post-workout recovery is a critical phase that significantly impacts an individual's fitness progress and overall health. After engaging in strenuous physical activity, the body undergoes various stressors, such as muscle tissue breakdown and depletion of energy stores. Proper recovery enables the body to repair and rebuild damaged tissues, replenish glycogen stores, and restore overall physiological balance. Neglecting post-workout recovery may lead to fatigue, increased risk of injury, and hindered performance in subsequent workouts. Adequate recovery strategies include nutrition, hydration, sleep, and active recovery techniques, ensuring that the body is well-prepared for future exercise sessions. Prioritizing post-workout recovery is fundamental for achieving optimal fitness results and sustaining a healthy exercise routine.

RELAXATION TECHNIQUES IN THE WATER

Water-based relaxation techniques offer a unique and effective approach to post-workout recovery. Immersing oneself in water provides buoyancy, reducing the impact on joints and muscles. This gentle environment facilitates relaxation and enhances circulation, aiding in the removal of metabolic waste products accumulated during exercise. Water-based relaxation may involve activities such as swimming, water aerobics, or simple floating exercises. The hydrostatic pressure of water also promotes improved blood circulation, reducing inflammation and promoting a sense of well-being. Additionally, the calming effect of water contributes to mental relaxation, reducing stress and promoting a positive mindset. Incorporating relaxation techniques in the water into a recovery routine provides a refreshing and holistic approach to fostering physical and mental well-being.

CHAPTER ELEVEN

TROUBLESHOOTING TYPICAL PROBLEMS

DEALING WITH MUSCLE CRAMPS

Muscle cramps are a common issue that can disrupt various physical activities, including exercise routines. These sudden, involuntary contractions of muscles can be caused by dehydration, electrolyte imbalances, or overuse. One effective way to deal with muscle cramps is to ensure proper hydration. Dehydrated muscles are more prone to cramping, so maintaining adequate fluid intake is crucial. Additionally, replenishing electrolytes, such as potassium, magnesium, and calcium, can help prevent imbalances that contribute to cramps.

Stretching before and after workouts are another strategy to reduce the likelihood of muscle cramps. Incorporating dynamic stretches into warm-ups and static stretches into cool-downs can enhance flexibility and minimize muscle tightness. Furthermore, avoiding overexertion and gradually increasing exercise intensity can prevent muscle fatigue, a common precursor to cramping. In cases where cramps do occur, gently massaging and stretching the affected muscle, along with applying heat or cold packs, can provide relief.

OVERCOMING PLATEAUS

Plateaus in fitness progress can be frustrating, but they are a natural part of any fitness journey. Overcoming plateaus requires a strategic approach that involves adjusting workout routines and focusing on key aspects of fitness. One effective method is to vary exercise routines regularly. The body tends to adapt to repetitive exercises, leading to diminished results. Introducing new exercises, changing workout intensity, or incorporating cross-training can shock the body and stimulate further progress.

Nutritional adjustments also play a crucial role in overcoming plateaus.

Ensuring a balanced diet with the right mix of macronutrients and micronutrients provides the energy needed for optimal performance. Additionally, paying attention to recovery is essential. Sufficient rest and quality sleep allow the body to repair and grow stronger. Adequate recovery time can help break through plateaus by preventing overtraining and reducing the risk of injury.

Setting realistic goals and tracking progress is another key aspect of overcoming plateaus. Regularly reassessing fitness goals and celebrating small achievements can provide motivation and direction. Seeking guidance from fitness professionals or trainers can offer valuable insights and personalized strategies to overcome specific plateaus.

INJURY PREVENTION IN WATER AEROBICS

Water aerobics is a low-impact exercise that provides numerous health benefits, but like any physical activity, it comes with the risk of injury. Proper injury prevention strategies are essential for ensuring a safe and enjoyable water aerobics experience. One fundamental aspect is warming up before diving into the main workout. Gentle water-based stretches and movements prepare the muscles and joints for more intense exercise, reducing the risk of strains or sprains.

Maintaining proper form during water aerobics is crucial for injury prevention. The buoyancy of water can sometimes mask improper technique, leading to overuse injuries. Attending classes or working with a certified instructor can help participants learn and maintain correct form. It's also important to listen to the body and avoid pushing beyond individual limits, especially for those with pre-existing conditions.

Investing in appropriate footwear for water aerobics can provide additional support and stability. Water shoes with non-slip soles help prevent slips and falls, minimizing the risk of injuries in and around the pool.

CHAPTER TWELVE

COMBINING WATER AEROBICS WITH OTHER FITNESS ACTIVITIES

CROSS-TRAINING STRATEGIES

Combining water aerobics with other fitness activities offers a holistic approach to overall well-being, incorporating cross-training strategies to enhance physical fitness and achieve a more comprehensive workout routine. Cross-training involves engaging in a variety of exercises to target different muscle groups and energy systems, promoting overall strength, flexibility, and cardiovascular health. Water aerobics, with its low-impact nature, provides an excellent platform for cross-training, allowing individuals to diversify their workouts without putting excessive strain on joints and muscles.

INTEGRATING LAND-BASED WORKOUTS

Integrating land-based workouts into a water aerobics routine introduces a dynamic element to the fitness regimen. Transitioning between aquatic exercises and traditional land-based workouts, such as strength training or cardiovascular exercises, challenges the body in various ways. The buoyancy of water reduces the impact on joints, making it an ideal environment for individuals with joint issues or those recovering from injuries. The resistance provided by water adds intensity to strength training, leading to increased muscle engagement and improved overall conditioning.

BALANCING EXERCISE REGIMENS

Balancing exercise regimens becomes a key focus when combining water aerobics with other fitness activities. Achieving balance involves addressing different aspects of fitness, including cardiovascular endurance, strength, flexibility, and stability. Water aerobics, with its focus on resistance and fluid movements, complements land-based activities by targeting muscle groups not always engaged during traditional workouts. By incorporating a mix of aerobic exercises, strength training, and flexibility routines, individuals can develop a well-rounded fitness routine that promotes overall health and longevity.

The combination of water aerobics and land-based workouts also allows for versatility in training intensity. Water provides natural resistance, requiring the body to work harder to move through it. This increased resistance contributes to improved cardiovascular fitness and muscle endurance. On land, individuals can further challenge themselves with higher-impact activities to enhance bone density and promote weight-bearing exercise benefits. Striking a balance between low-impact water exercises and higher-impact land-based activities fosters a comprehensive approach to fitness, catering to different fitness levels and preferences.

Moreover, the social aspect of water aerobics can be seamlessly integrated into land-based activities. Group fitness classes, whether in the pool or on solid ground, foster a sense of community and support. Engaging in a variety of workouts with others creates a motivating environment, encouraging individuals to stay consistent with their fitness routines. This integration of social interaction enhances the overall well-being aspect of fitness, addressing not only the physical but also the mental and emotional components of a healthy lifestyle.

Combining water aerobics with other fitness activities through cross-training strategies, integrating land-based workouts, and balancing exercise regimens provides a holistic approach to physical fitness. This comprehensive approach targets various aspects of health, promoting overall well-being and creating a versatile and enjoyable fitness routine. Whether in the water or on land, the integration of diverse exercises enhances the effectiveness of the workout, catering to individual preferences and accommodating different fitness levels.

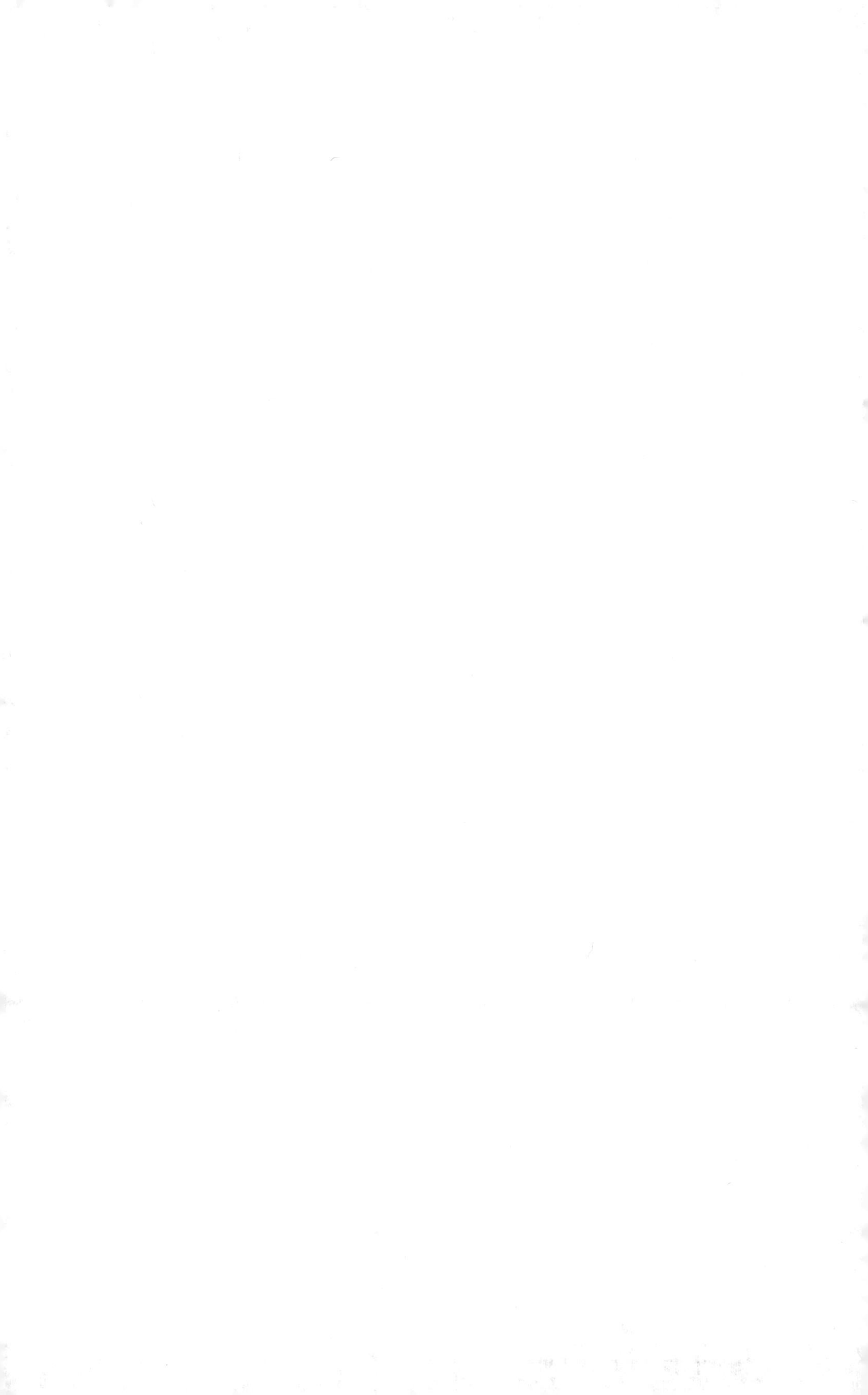

9 798325 782022